D0625781

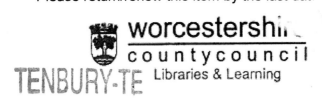

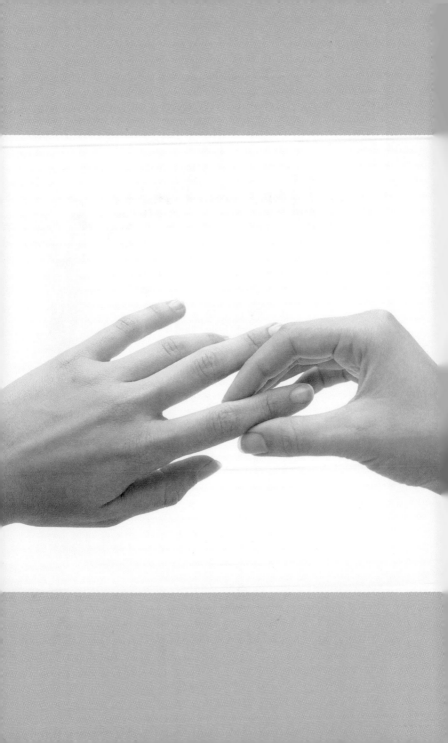

reflexology
therapies & techniques for well-being

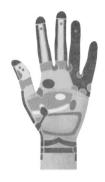

BERYL CRANE

DUNCAN BAIRD PUBLISHERS

LONDON

reflexology
Beryl Crane

To the memory of my beloved husband Reg,
who supported me totally in every aspect of
my work. And to my fellow colleagues who
have worked tirelessly alongside me in the
quest to get reflexology recognised at the
professional level it deserves.

First published in the United Kingdom and
Ireland in 2005 by
Duncan Baird Publishers Ltd
Sixth Floor, Castle House
75–76 Wells Street, London W1T 3QH

This edition published in 2010

Conceived, created and designed by
Duncan Baird Publishers Ltd

Copyright © Duncan Baird Publishers
2005, 2010
Text copyright © Beryl Crane 2005, 2010
Commissioned artwork copyright ©
Duncan Baird Publishers 2005, 2010
Commissioned photography copyright ©
Duncan Baird Publishers 2005, 2010
For copyright of agency photographs
see p.128, which is to be regarded as an
extension of this copyright.

The right of Beryl Crane to be identified as
the Author of this text has been asserted in
accordance with the Copyright, Designs and
Patents Act of 1988.

Managing Designer: Manisha Patel
Designer: Allan Sommerville
Managing Editor: Julia Charles
Editor: Rebecca Miles
Picture Research: Julia Ruxton
Commissioned Photography: Matthew Ward

British Library Cataloguing-in-Publication
Data:
A CIP record for this book is available from
the British Library.

ISBN: 978-1-84483-877-6

10 9 8 7 6 5 4 3 2 1

Typeset in Filosofia and Son Kern
Colour reproduction by Scanhouse, Malaysia
Printed in Malaysia for Imago

Publisher's note:
The information in this book is not intended
as a substitute for professional medical
advice and treatment. If you are pregnant or
are suffering from any medical conditions
or health problems, it is recommended that
you consult a medical professional before
following any of the advice or practice
suggested in this book. Duncan Baird
Publishers, or any other persons who have
been involved in working on this publication,
cannot accept responsibility for any injuries
or damage incurred as a result of following
the information, exercises or therapeutic
techniques contained in this book.

Abbreviations used throughout this book:
CE Common Era (the equivalent of AD)
BCE Before the Common Era (the equivalent
of BC)

CONTENTS

INTRODUCTION

Throughout the history of mankind, the power of touch has been used as a restorative; to bring back health and strength after illness and to promote general well-being. Today, the laying on of hands is used in many therapies and cultures to prevent illness and to bring about cures. This book will show you how to maintain good physical and emotional health, for yourself and for others, through the healing touch therapy of reflexology.

Reflexology is a totally holistic non-invasive natural therapy, which aims to treat imbalances within the body and enhance its innate ability to heal itself. The practice is based on the principle that every part of the body is interdependent and that the body needs to maintain a state of balance for optimum energy flow and health. With reflexology, this balance is achieved by applying pressure to points on the feet and hands that correspond to every organ in the body. By pressing these "reflex points", you can stimulate or sedate the nerve pathways linking the points to the corresponding organs. This encourages the various body parts and systems to work optimally, both individually and as part of the whole.

Reflexology, like many touch therapies, is based on the theory that, for total health, the body's energy must flow around it unimpeded. Any physical or emotional imbalances can block this flow and disrupt the body's inner equilibrium. Reflexology is a practical healing method, which produces various responses according to the needs of the patient's body. It also induces a state of calm and relaxation, alleviating harmful stress and tension.

This book explains the origins and theories of reflexology and shows you how to prepare for practice. It presents basic sessions for the feet and hands and explores how reflexology treatment can be used on particular body systems and ailments. My vision is to see reflexology accepted and practised worldwide at a professional level, so that all may benefit from its preventative and curative properties. Whether you are new to reflexology or an established practitioner, I sincerely hope that you enjoy reading this book and will learn something from the many years of clinical experience portrayed within its pages.

origins and basics

Reflexology is an art and a science based upon the principle that there are reflex points on the hands and feet corresponding to all the organs of the body. It was developed in the early 20th century by doctors in the United States and Europe who were studying the role of reflex actions within the nervous system. As reflexology theory progressed, parallels were drawn with aspects of ancient medical traditions from Egypt, Greece, India and, in particular, China. Today, many reflexologists draw on parts of these traditions to help inform their holistic approach to practice.

Now well-established internationally, reflexology supports nature by regulating any imbalances in the body and encouraging the best conditions for the maintenance of peak health. As well as improving many symptoms for patients suffering from a particular illness, regular reflexology benefits those in good health by maintaining just that and by working as a marvellous preventative.

In this chapter we look at the beginnings of reflexology and the theories upon which it is based. We explain how it works and offer advice on how and where to start, including practical information on preparing for a session and establishing a therapeutic relationship with a patient, in order to equip you with the tools and confidence to begin.

HOW REFLEXOLOGY WORKS

Although the therapeutic benefits of reflexology are well documented and countless case histories attest to its pain-relieving properties, there is as yet no concise explanation as to how it actually works. However, theories abound – many based on scientific facts concerning brain and nervous-system function. It is an area of science about which there is still much to learn. The creation of government-funded specialist centres offering reflexology to help conditions such as pain, multiple sclerosis and cancer, stands as a good counter-argument to those in the medical establishment who remain sceptical.

By definition, reflexology is associated with the role of reflex actions within the body. A reflex is an involuntary activity brought about by a simple nervous circuit, without consciousness being involved. Removing a hand from a hot surface is one example. A sensory cell on the surface of the skin reacts by sending a signal along the nerve fibre to the central nervous system, which then transmits a signal to another nerve cell which is also activated. This action is enough to cause a muscle to contract or to increase the secretory function of a gland.

The workings of a reflex action demonstrate the law of nerves which states that they respond to energy, whether mechanically or electrically excited. The stimulation of nerve cells, or reflex points, on the feet and hands during a reflexology session transmits energy along nerve pathways and helps to regulate this energy flow throughout the body and its various organs. This regulation, or balancing, of energy flow around the body via the nervous system helps create the ideal environment for the body to rebalance or begin to heal itself of a host of ailments. Reflexology is also believed to stimulate the release of endorphins in the brain – natural chemicals which have pain-relieving qualities. In addition, the deep sense of relaxation normally felt by a patient after reflexology has the effect of reducing muscle tension and relieving anxiety and stress. This all feeds into the upward spiral of general physical and emotional well-being that a holistic therapy such as reflexology seeks to promote.

HISTORICAL BEGINNINGS

Evidence of healing therapies using pressure techniques or massage can be found in past civilizations such as those from Egypt, Greece, India and China.

The earliest reference comes from the tomb of Ankhm'ahor in Saqqara, Egypt, and dates back to the Sixth Dynasty (2345–2184 BCE). This tomb is known as the "physician's tomb", because of the many medical scenes depicted in wonderful detail on its walls. One such scene shows reflexology-style treatments being given on the hands and feet of seated figures (see right). The hieroglyphics above the images have one figure (the patient) saying, "Make these give strength", and another responding, "I will do to thy pleasure, sovereign".

In Ancient Greece, the renowned physician, Hippocrates (460–377 BCE), known today as the "father of medicine", recommended a holistic system of healthcare which incorporated diet, fresh air and exercise. He also advocated massage or rubbing an area as therapeutic relaxation and pain relief.

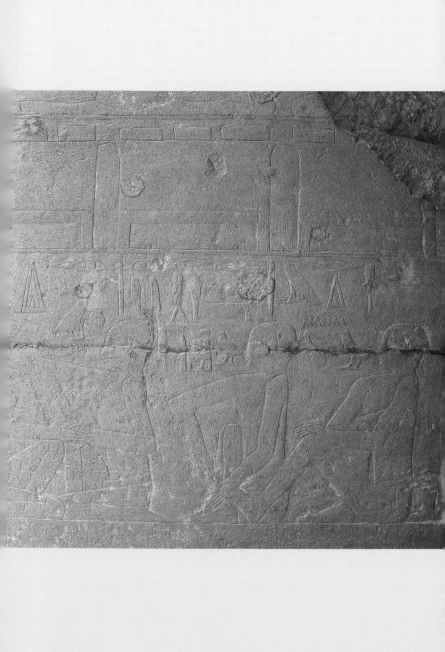

Traditional Chinese Medicine

The system of medicine practised in China for thousands of years, and still important today, is known as Traditional Chinese Medicine (TCM). This is the system perhaps most closely associated with modern reflexology because its central theory of "Qi", or "Ch'i", focuses on a balance of energy flow around the body as a way to maintain health and prevent illness. Qi is described as a vital, unseen, nutritive inner energy or force that must

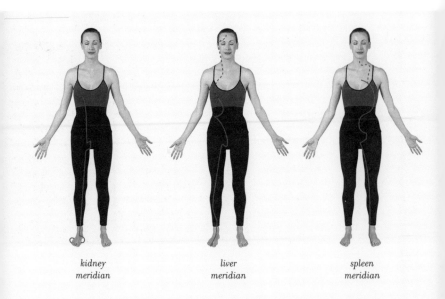

kidney
meridian

liver
meridian

spleen
meridian

flow without a blockage through the body. Illness is seen as an imbalance of this energy.

Qi flows around the body along channels or pathways called meridians, and these are manipulated by a range of pressure techniques to keep the Qi moving and to remedy any imbalance or stagnation. There are twelve major meridians within the body, each one named after an associated key organ or part of the body (see below and pp.16–17). These meridians and their organs or

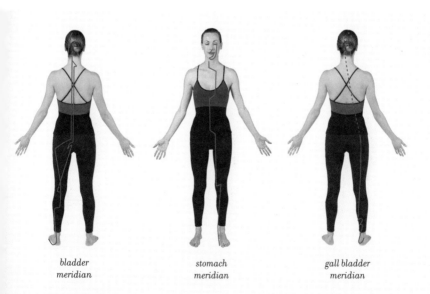

bladder meridian

stomach meridian

gall bladder meridian

body parts are divided into two groups – the Yin and Yang groups – in accordance with another basic Chinese philosophy, the principle of Yin and Yang.

Yin and Yang are two opposite but complementary principles which govern everything in the universe. Their balanced interaction is necessary to maintain harmony in all things, including bodily health. The two forces are never static – they balance one another and regulate the whole organism. Yin is represented by the

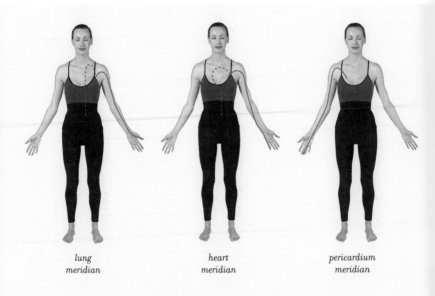

lung
meridian

heart
meridian

pericardium
meridian

negative, dark and feminine, while Yang is the positive, bright and masculine. Within the body, the Yin parts – kidneys, liver, spleen, lung, heart and pericardium – are all solid, and the Yang parts – bladder, stomach, gall bladder, large intestine, small intestine and "triple burner" (comprising the respiratory, digestive and pelvic areas) – are all hollow.

The Yin and Yang philosophy in regard to meridians bears striking parallels with two key complementary

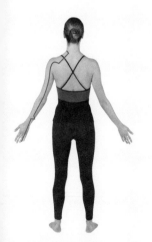
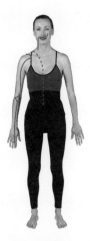
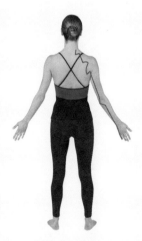

triple burner
meridian

large intestine
meridian

small intestine
meridian

parts of the body's nervous system: the Sympathetic and the Parasympathetic nervous systems. The nerves of the Sympathetic system are activated when the body needs to create the conditions required for physical exertion, and the Parasympathetic nerves dominate when the body needs to create conditions conducive to rest, sleep and digestion. Similarly, reactions to the stimulation of the Yang meridians are said to be positive and to represent activity, while reactions to the stimulation of the Yin meridians are typically calming.

Today, the pressure techniques based on TCM that are used to manipulate the meridians include acupressure, acupuncture and shiatsu massage. The meridians traverse the whole body and each one has a series of pressure points along its trajectory which are worked to regulate the flow of the Qi and to benefit the associated organ or body part. One of the points on each meridian is known as a "source point". This is located at a particular place in its trajectory, usually near the ankle or the wrist. If there is any disease or disorder of the meridian's key organ or body part, an abnormal reaction, such as a swelling, some discolouration, or varicose veins, may be evident at the source point.

The meridian points on the extremities of the body (the feet and the hands) are particularly powerful because the Qi here, at the starting or terminal point of the meridian, is barely skin deep. Working various points elsewhere along the meridian is still highly effective but achieves a slower response. These points in the hands and feet are the ones that some reflexology practitioners incorporate into their treatment sessions today.

TCM and its branch of Meridian Theory are both thoroughly comprehensive medical systems with their own theories and philosophies regarding diagnostic methods and practice. There are many intriguing parallels to be drawn between these systems and reflexology, and it is entirely in keeping with reflexology's holistic approach to health that we should explore any links between the therapies. However, reflexology was developed quite separately from any Eastern medical tradition, by an American doctor working in the early 20th century on a theory he called "Zone Therapy".

THE ZONE CONCEPT

Zone Therapy, the system upon which modern reflexology is based, was developed in the early 20th century by an American doctor, William Fitzgerald (1872–1942) from Hartford, Connecticut. A graduate of the University of Vermont, Fitzgerald first worked in Boston City Hospital before two periods abroad, at specialist Ear, Nose and Throat hospitals in London and Vienna. He went on to become a senior nose and throat surgeon at St. Francis Hospital in Hartford, and it was here that he first made public his work on Zone Therapy.

It was Fitzgerald's belief that the human body could be divided into ten longitudinal zones, five on each side of the body's median line. Each zone extends from the centre of one of the toes, runs up through the body to the top of the head and out along the arm to the fingers or thumbs. The zones are numbered one to five on both the left and right sides of the body, radiating out from the middle (see right). Fitzgerald referred to the zone lines as ten invisible currents of energy running through the body, with each line representing the centre of the respective zone. Each zone could be treated by working on either the feet or the hands.

He found that if pressure was applied to any bony part of the body within a particular zone, especially on the hands and feet, body organs elsewhere in the same zone were affected positively. Pain caused by an injury somewhere in the zone was relieved and, if pressure was

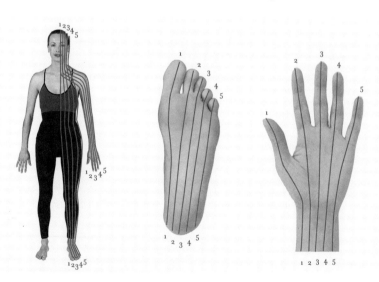

applied firmly enough, a type of localized anaesthesia would occur sometimes causing the injury or problem to disappear completely. Fitzgerald used clamps, combs and pegs, mainly on the hands, to create the desired anaesthetic effect throughout the whole zone.

In 1917, Fitzgerald and a colleague, Dr. Edwin Bowers, published *Zone Therapy, or Relieving Pain at Home*, a pioneering volume still much used by reflexologists today. In it Fitzgerald also referred to "anatomical correspondences". This refers to the pairing of corresponding parts of the body in terms of reflexology practice for example, hand and foot, wrist and ankle, elbow and knee, upper arm and thigh, shoulder and hip. If, when treating a patient, a particular area is too sore or damaged to work on for any reason, the reflexologist can work on the corresponding area with good effect. In reflexology today, these are termed the "cross reflexes".

Fitzgerald's book on Zone Therapy was followed by several others, written by medical colleagues and students of the great doctor. One such person was Dr. Joseph Shelby-Riley who published twelve books on the subject between 1919 and 1942. One of Shelby-Riley's students was a young therapist named Eunice Ingham who went on to become a pivotal figure in early reflexology. In the 1930s, Ingham built on Fitzgerald's original zone theory, defining three significant developments that had a major impact on the practical application of the therapy.

First, she introduced usage of the compression method known as "alternating pressure", favouring it over Fitzgerald's application of constant pressure during treatment. This was more of a "press-release" action by the thumb or finger, travelling along the skin in a caterpillar-like movement, but without ever losing contact. Ingham felt that this stimulated healing to a far greater effect than the "numbing" technique used previously. Second, she advocated working primarily on the foot reflexes (above those of the hand) as she found these more sensitive and, therefore, more effective as a treatment.

Finally, and perhaps most important of all, Ingham introduced a detailed foot map showing how the position of the organs of the body are reflected on the feet. "Reflex maps" of the feet and hands have been refined over subsequent decades, and should replicate the anatomical arrangement of the body, marking the neurological reflexes to the corresponding organs. In effect the feet and hands act as a micro-system of the body. More than 70 reflex areas have now been identified (see maps on pages 120–124).

In addition, reflexologists today work within four transverse divisions of the feet and hands, which are similarly reflected in the corresponding zones of the body. These are known as the "transverse zones" or "guide lines" and were introduced later. They are used as an additional guide for practitioners as to where to work, and they complement the more detailed reflex maps. Each body part or system that a reflexologist may wish to treat will always fall within one of these transverse zones which, again, correspond anatomically to a body map. The four zones are divided by imaginary lines (see right) which are described as the shoulder line, diaphragm line, waist line and hip line.

The area above the shoulder line (on the feet and hands) refers to parts of the head and neck; the area between the shoulder and diaphragm lines refers to the upper parts of the body such as the chest, lungs, breast and heart; the area between the diaphragm and waist lines covers the middle section of the body, including such parts as the liver, gall bladder, kidney, stomach, pancreas, spleen and solar plexus; and the area between the waist and hip lines refers to the intestines, bladder, and pelvic, buttock and lumbar areas.

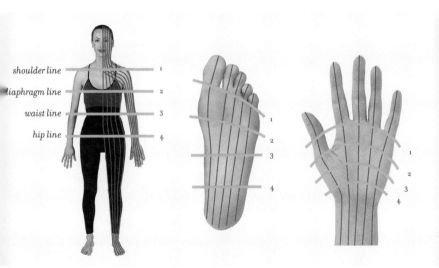

shoulder line — 1
diaphragm line — 2
waist line — 3
hip line — 4

WHERE TO BEGIN

Before embarking on any reflexology treatment, on yourself or others, there are several factors to consider to enable you to maximize its healing potential. You need to choose whether to work on the hands or feet; be aware of any special precautions needed on account of your or a patient's general health; and prepare yourself and your surroundings for a comfortable, therapeutic session.

Feet or hands?

Without a doubt, foot reflexology is the most powerful application of the therapy and pressure on the reflex points of the feet stimulates the nerve pathways and organs more vigorously than working the hands. There are certain circumstances, however, in which treating the feet may not be advisable and hand treatments are by far the better option.

If a patient is seriously ill, avoid treating the feet as the therapy's generally detoxifying effect could stimulate the release of more toxins around the body than usual (see pp.38–9). Also, refrain from treating the feet if the patient is suffering from any disorder or injury of the foot, such as a fracture or broken bone, an ulcer, gout or any wound which could be painful if touched or cause cross-infection. In addition conditions such as rheumatism or severe arthritis may make it too painful to treat the feet. If you are in any doubt about treating the feet for any reason, seek advice from an experienced accredited practitioner before you begin.

Hand reflexology is an effective and often convenient alternative to working on the feet. Treatment can be given anywhere – there are no socks or shoes to remove and it can be less intimidating and very soothing for a nervous patient. It is suitable for everyone from new-borns to the elderly and infirm, and for all of the types of cases mentioned above apart from rheumatoid arthritis where there is bad deformity of the hands. However, some people may not be comfortable having their hands touched, perhaps feeling it somehow invades their personal space, so it is important that you tailor each treatment session appropriately for each individual patient.

Contraindications

Reflexology is a holistic, non-invasive, safe therapy, which does not attempt to treat medical disorders, rather it redresses any imbalances within the body and creates the optimum conditions for the body to heal itself. There are some unsubstantiated myths concerning possible side-effects of reflexology saying, for example, that it can make a medical condition worse, cause cancer to spread or induce a heart attack. It cannot. However, as with any therapy, sensible precautions should be taken before treating some patients:

- Do not work on someone suffering from a contagious disease because of the risk of cross-infection.
- If a patient is about to undertake medical tests, it is inadvisable to work as reflexology could improve their immediate general condition and distort the outcome.
- If there is excessive sensitivity (or a lack of sensitivity, as in the disease neuropathy which affects the peripheral nerves), care should be taken not to cause bruising when applying pressure.

- Do not treat a patient suffering from thrombosis or DVT until the condition has been stabilized. Reflexology improves the circulation but it is advisable to get the consent of the patient's doctor before treatment.
- Before reflexology treatment for a patient suffering from cancer, it is advisable to complete some specialized training for work in this field.
- In the case of pregnancy, it is helpful to have tutorials from a trained midwife to gain an understanding of the whole birth process – from conception to delivery – so you can adapt your treatment program accordingly. Many practitioners do not treat pregnant women because of the danger of litigation, so it is imperative to work within your limitations. Reflexology is wonderful for pain relief in labour, but it must be given in agreement with the patient's medical team.

When treating any patient suffering from a medical disorder, it is essential to have an understanding of the condition and to adapt reflexology treatment, including the use of an appropriate level of pressure, accordingly.

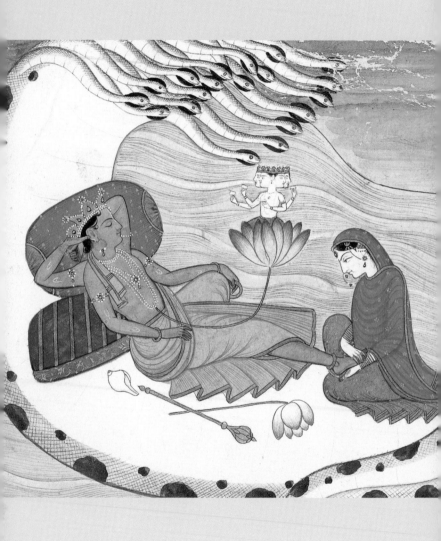

As is the human body, so is the cosmic body
As is the human mind, so is the cosmic mind
As is the microcosm, so is the macrocosm
As is the atom, so is the universe

THE UPANISHADS
(8TH–4TH CENTURY BCE)

Preparing for a session

Whether practising reflexology in your own home or at the home of a patient, it is important to create a suitable environment for treatment. The place where you work should be peaceful, private and comfortable, perhaps with some quiet relaxing music playing in the background. A typical reflexology session may well last for up to an hour so it is vital to ensure the comfort of both patient and practitioner.

The room you use should be well-lit, well-ventilated, scrupulously clean and pleasantly warm. Patients should be seated on a suitable reclining chair or bench that is covered with clean linens and paper or fresh towels at each session. Pillows can be placed behind the head and back, and under the knees so that the patient is in a semi-recumbent position. Take care that they aren't bent into a "U" shape at all because, during the course of a session, this could divert blood flow and cause congestion in the pathways of the abdominal organs.

When working, the practitioner should be seated comfortably, with a straight back, preferably on an adjustable low stool, so that the feet or hands of the patient are at chest height, allowing for clear eye contact. There is no need to use oils or lotions during treatment as these can cause the hands to slip off the reflexes. If you really wish to use talcum powder, keep this to an absolute minimum: when inhaled, the dust produced can irritate allergies and may cause respiratory problems.

Before starting reflexology at a session, always make an assessment of the patient's general demeanour so that you can tailor the treatment accordingly. You can learn a great deal about a person's state of health just by observing their body language when they enter the room. Pay special attention to posture, breathing and tone of voice, and look out for clues, such as uneven wear and tear of shoes, that may indicate an imbalance in the body (see also pp.44–7). If you are treating someone for the first time, take a full case history to inform your approach.

Once the preliminary preparations for a session are complete, it is important to establish a therapeutic relationship between patient and practitioner so that the patient can gain the maximum benefit from reflexology.

Establishing a therapeutic relationship

One of the keys to the success of a touch therapy such as reflexology is for the patient and practitioner to establish and maintain a therapeutic relationship.

As you are the practitioner, preparation for this relationship should begin with you, and you need to equip yourself physically, mentally and emotionally to give treatment. Make sure you are sitting comfortably in a relaxed position before you start – an incorrect working position can cause repetitive strain injuries on your hands and shoulders. Mentally and emotionally you should be in a relaxed state – any tension could adversely affect your work. Try a short relaxation exercise or take a few deep breaths before you begin.

Take a holistic approach to reflexology and its practice and share this with your patient where possible. Be aware of other therapies (such as aromatherapy massage) that may complement the treatment. You might discuss lifestyle choices, such as diet and exercise, that could highlight an underlying cause of a patient's illness or imbalance. People do not become ill overnight, and many health problems could be avoided if we all became more aware of behaviour patterns and lifestyle issues, and how these may impact on our health.

Endeavour to be a good communicator – make sure you are able both to give and to receive information effectively. Speak clearly but gently, and listen actively so that you encourage your patient to communicate openly with you. Before starting a session, be sure to discuss the aims of the treatment so that you are both happy with all aspects of it.

Perhaps the most important facet of a therapeutic relationship is the ability to cultivate empathy with a fellow human being. Our emotions – joy, fear or anger, to name a few – can cause changes to the internal organs and their functions: for example, the heartbeat, breathing or glandular secretion may speed up or slow down. To be able to identify, recognise and comprehend some of the emotions and feelings that may be causing an imbalance in a patient, and to really empathise with them, will help you to build and maintain a valuable therapeutic relationship.

The basic pressure techniques

There are many different pressure techniques used in reflexology but the traditional and most commonly used are the moving technique of alternating pressure (see p.23), the stationary technique, and the techniques that work more deeply such as "hooking" and "knuckling". Of these, the moving technique of alternating pressure, often referred to as "finger-" or "thumb-walking", is used most widely by reflexologists. It is a straightforward and effective technique, and ideal for working many of the larger reflex areas.

The smaller reflexes, by their nature, need to be more precisely located, and these often require a stationary or rotating technique where the thumb or finger is not lifted from the skin.

To work more deeply, you may use a hooking technique, where you apply your thumb in a bent position, pushing in and hooking back. You can also rock on the spot using the thumb in this hooked position. Alternatively, you can use the knuckle for deep work, in either a stationary, moving or sweeping action.

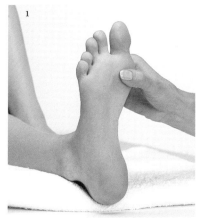

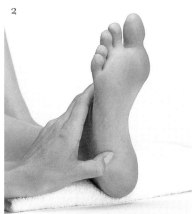

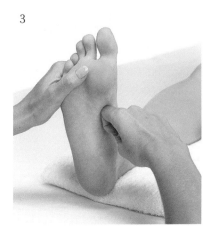

As well as the alternating pressure technique, the stationary technique (1), "hooking" technique (2) and "knuckling" technique (3) can all be used when working on the various reflexes of the foot.

POSSIBLE REACTIONS TO TREATMENT

Various responses to reflexology treatment may occur during or after a session. These relate to the stimulation of the nervous system by work on the reflexes and to the movement and elimination of toxins in the body. This shows that the treatment is working and achieving its aim of regulating and rebalancing the body systems and their functions. Reactions that the patient may experience during treatment include:

- Sweating of the palms as tension eases
- Coughing, laughing, crying or sighing deeply as pent-up emotions are released
- Twitching or tingling in the limbs
- A feeling of movement, sudden cramp, or an electric-type shock up the zone being worked, or a feeling of warmth in the corresponding area, and sometimes on the opposite side of the body
- Great fatigue with an overwhelming desire to sleep
- The disappearance of pain and discomfort

The patient should note down any reactions that occur following a treatment session so that you can make a full evaluation of the session and adapt any future treatments as necessary. It is quite common for reactions to be slightly exacerbated in the first 24 hours after a session. Post-treatment reactions may include:

- Flu-like symptoms with aches and pains
- The appearance of skin rashes, spots or pimples
- Yellow or greenish sputum from a respiratory tract infection often becomes clear
- Feeling lethargic for approximately 48 hours
- Increased thirst, wind or flatulence
- Increase in the frequency and ease of bowel movements with an increased flow of urine
- An overall sense of well-being, with increased energy and the disappearance of tension and anxiety
- Improvement in sleeping patterns
- Disappearance of pain and discomfort with more mobility in the joints for increasing lengths of time after each of a series of treatment sessions

No bird soars too high, if he soars with his own wings.

WILLIAM BLAKE

(1757– 1827)

Though we travel the world over to find the beautiful,
we must carry it within us or we find it not.

RALPH WALDO EMERSON

(1803– 1882)

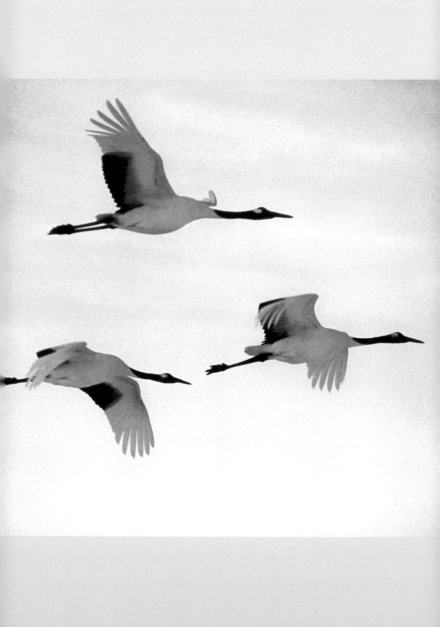

foot reflexology

The foot is an architectural wonder. It contains 26 bones, 107 ligaments and 19 main muscles, all served by nerves which cover every area and surface. In reflexology, applying pressure to these nerves transmits energy and sends electrical messages around the body, stimulating or sedating the parts of the body that correspond to the relevant reflexes.

This chapter takes you through a basic reflexology session for the feet. We look at how you should first examine the feet for possible indications of illness or imbalances in the body, and the correct ways in which to hold the feet when working. Next there is a section on warming and relaxing techniques for you to apply to your patient at the start of a session, and a comprehensive step-by-step guide to treatment, covering all the major organs of the body, detailing the locations of the relevant reflexes and how best to work them. We finish with some advice on basic foot care and suggested exercises to keep the feet supple and to further stimulate the reflex areas.

The information given focuses on applying reflexology to another person, but it is equally valid for self-treatment. All you need do is adapt how you hold the foot and apply pressure so that you can work comfortably and you will soon be benefitting from the enhanced health and well-being that reflexology provides.

INTERPRETING THE FOOT

Before beginning a session of foot reflexology, the practitioner should spend some time analyzing the patient's feet and interpreting various physical characteristics. This is with a view to building a picture of the patient's constitution and any problems that may be causing an imbalance within it. It is important, too, to consider the feet in conjunction with a general assessment of the whole patient, taking into consideration mood and any other physical or emotional characteristics that may give clues to a pre-existing condition or enforce a conclusion that you have drawn from looking at your patient's feet.

Observe your patient's posture as they enter the room, looking for any obvious physical imbalances, such as in the neck or lower back areas, that could be addressed by working the relevant reflexes. Listen carefully to your patient's breathing and speech – laboured breathing could indicate a respiratory problem; rapid breathing or speech can be a sign of stress; and deep sighing could indicate depression. Assessing such factors before giving reflexology to a patient provides helpful background information, and you may be surprised at just how many of your conclusions are borne out when you make a closer inspection of the feet.

The feet are a microcosm of the whole body and, in reflexology terms, an imaginary map of the body can be drawn on them, with the head lying at the end with the toes and the rest of the body working down toward the heel (see p.122–24). Interestingly, a person's feet also reflect their general build and body shape. For example, somebody with broad shoulders will have broad feet and someone who is tall and slim will have long, narrow feet.

When making your assessment of the feet, take a systematic approach:

• Compare the two inner ankle bones. If one looks higher than the other this shows that the hip on that side could be drawn up indicating spinal imbalances.
• The suppleness of the arches reflects the degree of flexibilty in the spine. If the arches are low or completely flat, the spine may be too rigid.

- Nails should be pink and healthy, showing a good nerve and blood supply.
- The great toe: any discoloration may indicate poor blood flow to the brain or problems in the head area. A deformed nail can cause the person to suffer headaches.
- The second toe: if hooked or leaning either way, the patient may suffer mouth, jaw, eye or ear problems.
- The third toe: any thickening of the nail may indicate ear or eye problems.
- The fourth toe: any enlargement could be indicative of shoulder or knee problems with a tendency to inflammation of the joints.
- The fifth toe: this often suffers physical deformity due to the mechanical action of shoes. Any undue pain or inflammation can indicate imbalances relating to the head, shoulder or spinal areas.
- Purple, red or mottled areas on the ball of the foot may indicate cardiovascular problems. An indentation or red area under the fifth toe beneath the diaphragm line on the left foot can be indicative of problems relating to the heart muscle.

• Pressure from tight footwear can create problems across the neck and shoulder area. In turn, these can radiate down through the spinal area, affecting nerve pathways and interrupting the flow of energy to all body parts.

Conclude your assessment of the feet by employing your sense of touch and gently feeling the feet all over. This will enable you to notice any deposits under the skin, or any changes of texture in the tissue. These signs may indicate an imbalance in that reflex point or zone.

Perhaps the most telling sign of an imbalance in a certain part of the body is indicated by a sensitive or sore spot somewhere on the feet. This also points to an imbalance in the corresponding part of the body and is referred to as a congested area. When stimulated, any painful or tender reflex reacts by releasing that congestion into the system, helping to re-establish a balanced energy flow around the nerve pathways of the body. However, if you are ever in any doubt about any unexplained sensitivity on the feet, be sure to refer your patient to their doctor for advice.

HOLDING THE FOOT

Supporting and holding the foot correctly during reflexology enables you to work freely and with optimum
effect. You can use various holding techniques to ensure
that the area being worked is covered effectively, and
that the patient remains relaxed and comfortable.

1 When working above the waist line (see p.25), on the
sole of the foot, hold the foot so that your thumb is on the
ball and your fingers are on the top of the foot. Gently pull
the foot toward you so that the toes aren't leaning back.

2 When working below the waist line, allow the patient's
heel to rest in the palm of your supporting hand, using
your thumb to steady the foot.

3 When working the top of the foot, make a fist with your
supporting hand. Place the thumb of your working hand
in between your fist and your patient's foot to stabilize
the fingers of your working hand, increasing accessibility.

4 When working on the sides of the foot, keep the foot as
straight as possible, adapting any holds accordingly.

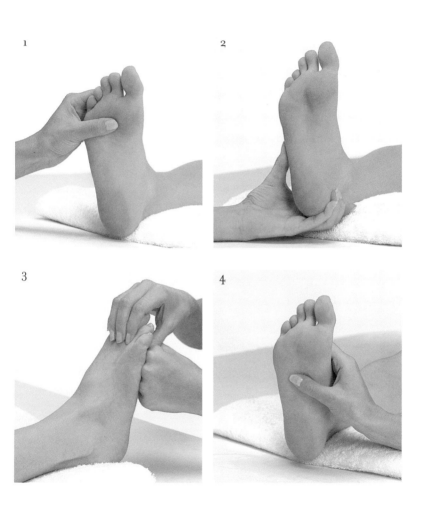

1

2

3

4

A BASIC SESSION FOR THE FEET

This section guides you through a basic reflexology session for the feet. First it presents some general warming and relaxing techniques and then shows you where to work on the foot to treat the major parts of the body, indicating some of the effects you might achieve.

Warming and relaxing techniques

These preliminary moves are designed to ease any muscular tension in the feet, relaxing them in prepara-tion for treatment. This has a knock-on effect of relaxing the whole body and putting the patient at ease at the beginning of the session. Any of these moves can be repeated at intervals during the session and again at the end of the treatment.

Strictly speaking, some of the methods described here may be classed as massage as they involve rubbing and kneading. They are, however, greatly beneficial to a reflexology session, enhancing treatment by improving the circulation of blood to any corresponding areas.

When making the initial contact with the foot, be very gentle as this will set the tone for the whole treatment session. Softly place your palms on the sole of each foot and hold for a moment. Next, place your thumbs on the solar plexus points (1) and apply unmoving pressure as the patient inhales and exhales slowly and deeply.

The following relaxation exercises may be applied in whichever order you find most comfortable:

Side friction Place palms on each side of the foot and slide your hands from toe to heel alternately (2).

1

2

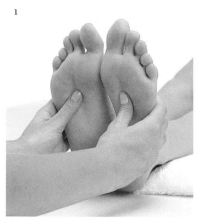

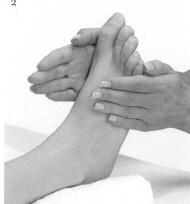

Side-to-side relaxation Move the foot alternately backward and forward without lifting the heel.

Ankle rotation Support the heel with one hand and encircle the base of the the great toe joint with the other. Rotate the foot in both directions several times.

Foot stretching Using the same support as ankle rotation, stretch the whole foot backward and forward.

Toe stretching and rotation Stretch and rotate each toe both ways, but be aware of arthritic joints.

Diaphragm relaxation Encircle the top of the foot with one hand flexing slightly toward the sole. Place the working thumb on the ball of the foot, pressing and lifting (3).

Metatarsal kneading Make a fist, knuckles in line with the base of the toes with the supporting hand on the top of the foot (4). Push and squeeze alternately.

Foot moulding Place your palms on the top and sole of the foot. Work them together as if rolling dough (5).

Ankle loosening Using the padded muscles at the base of your thumbs, place your hands in the depression on each side of the heel and move the foot from side to side (6). End by applying again the solar plexus pressure (1).

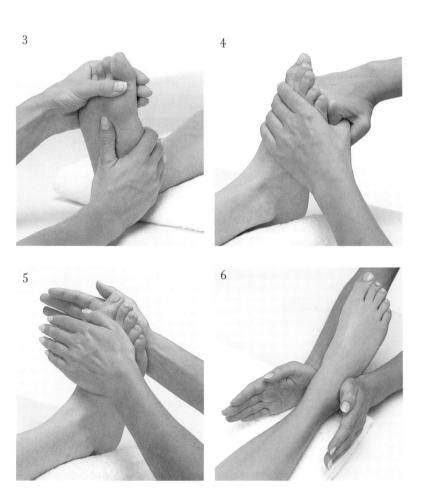

Working on the feet

The following pages offer a suggested order of work for treating the feet with reflexology. This basic foot session amounts to a full-body treatment for rebalancing the body, improving circulation and easing tension. We look at each aspect of the foot in turn and, within this, we identify groups of closely related organs and see their corresponding reflex areas marked on a map of the feet. Use these maps in conjunction with the reflex maps on pages 122–24 and the zone maps on pages 21 and 25. I also offer advice on the best way to work the reflexes.

You can apply reflexology to the feet in a variety of ways, using different pressure techniques (see p.36) and adapting treatment throughout the course of any particular session. You can work each reflex from different angles in a bid to ease congestion or tension in its corresponding body zone and organs. Although many body functions have reflex points on both feet, traditionally the right foot is treated first, and then the left. This enables a more systematic approach to covering all of the points required for a full reflexology treatment.

The soles of the feet

Lungs, heart and thymus The reflexes for these parts of the body are all found between the base of the toes and the diaphragm line on the soles of the feet. The lung reflex is the largest, reflecting the size of the lungs in the body itself. The thymus reflex is the small area on the medial edge of each foot. It is important to work this area in young children to promote healthy development or in patients suffering from any autoimmune disorder. The heart reflex is larger on the left foot than the right, reflecting the position of the heart within the body.

On both feet work from the medial (inner) to the lateral (outer) sides, applying pressure, with one hand, up and down the area in vertical strips. Then change hands and work back in the opposite direction.

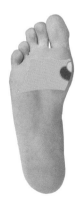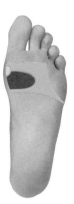

55

Brain, sinuses, eyes, ears, neck, thyroid and pituitary
The reflexes relating to the brain lie on the tips of the
first three toes, and the sinus reflexes cover the underneath of the same toes, from base to tip. The reflexes for
the eyes and ears are found just below the pads of the
second and third toes respectively. The area found at
the base of the first three toes, just below the shoulder
line, works the neck and thyroid reflexes. In addition,
this area acts as a "helper area" for the eyes and the
ears. The pituitary reflex is located in the middle of the
pad of the great toe.

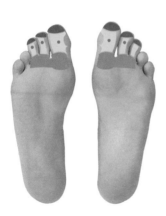

For the brain area, work
with thumb or index finger
in alternating steps, or use
the knuckle in a rolling
action. For the sinuses, eyes
and ears work in vertical
strips up or down each toe,
covering all sides. For the
neck and thyroid, work
horizontally. Apply firm
pressure to the pituitary,
eye and ear reflexes.

Liver, gall bladder, stomach, spleen and pancreas The larger of the two liver reflex areas is on the right foot, the smaller one on the left foot. Both areas are found between the waist and the diaphragm lines (see p.25). The small gall bladder reflex is found toward the bottom of the liver area on the right foot. The stomach reflex is in the same transverse zone, with the larger reflex area on the left foot. The spleen reflex can be found on the outer edge of the stomach reflex, on the left foot only, and the pancreas reflex is located a little above the waist line on both feet, with the larger area on the left foot.

To treat all of the reflexes marked, apply pressure in diagonal strips working in both directions. This is easier than working in horizontal bands as the skin remains taut. If there is a tender spot, apply pressure in circular rotations.

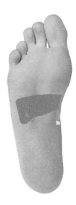
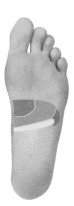

Ascending, transverse and descending colon, and small intestine The reflexes that relate to these parts of the body cover most of the area between the hip and the waist line (see p.25) on both feet. Treating them can be particularly beneficial to all aspects of the body's digestive system and process. In addition, work the ileocaecal valve, which connects the small and large intestines in the body, to further improve digestive function. This reflex can be found on the right foot, exactly on the heel line, about one thumb's breadth in from the lateral, or outer, edge.

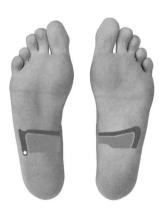

Apply pressure to the ileocaecal valve three times and work up the lateral edge of the right foot. Next, work all areas in horizontal lines, moving back and forth from the medial to the lateral sides of the feet. Then repeat the process working from the lateral to the medial sides.

Sigmoid colon, buttock and sciatic areas The sigmoid colon is the last part of the colon before the rectum. The associated reflex is found in a "V" shape descending just below the hip line (see p.25) on the left foot. Working this reflex can help with the defecation process and can also improve the symptoms of haemorrhoids. The reflexes relating to the buttocks cover a large area at the base of the heel on both feet. The reflex area corresponding to the sciatic nerve runs in a line across both feet at the top of the buttock reflex area, approximately midway between the base of the heel and the hip line.

On the left foot, work down from the descending colon reflex on the lateral side of the area with your right thumb, using alternating pressure. Continue to the base of the sigmoid colon reflex, and up the other side of this reflex. Then work in horizontal strips across the buttock and sciatic areas on both feet.

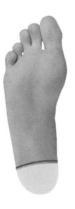
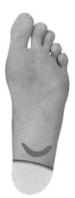

Bladder, ureters, adrenal glands and kidneys The bladder reflexes are located on the slightly raised rounded area on the medial, or inner, side of both feet which traverses the hip line (see p.25). The kidney reflex areas lie just above the waist line in the second longitudinal zone (see p.21). The reflexes for the ureters (the tubes that convey the urine from the kidneys to the bladder) run in a line between the kidney and bladder reflexes on both feet, and the adrenal gland reflexes lie approximately two finger breadths below the diaphragm line, just above the kidney reflex.

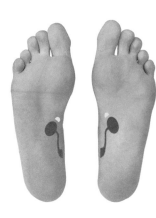

Using the thumb, make tiny steps on the bladder reflex. Continue up the medial edge of the foot, working the ureters, to the adrenal gland. Rotate on this point. Return to the bladder, work up to the waist line and across to the kidney reflex. Apply unmoving pressure to this point, rotating the foot down onto the thumb with the other hand.

The tops of the feet

Facial area The main reflex points for the facial area are found on the front of the great toe. They include the reflexes for the nose, mouth and throat, the windpipe (trachea) and the important trigeminal nerves which serve the entire facial area. Reflexes for the teeth can also be accessed on the front of the second and third toes. Also, in addition to the reflex points for the neck and thyroid found on the soles of the feet (see p.56), there are further points for these areas located on the top of each foot at the base of the first three toes.

To cover the reflexes for the nose, mouth, throat, trachea and trigeminal nerves, work with your index finger in tiny horizontal strips from the nail bed down to the base of the great toe. For the neck and thyroid reflexes, work horizontally across the area from the medial edge to the second and third toes, and then back again.

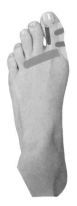
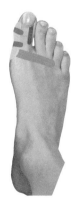

Lungs and upper part of the lymphatic system Reflex areas for the lungs are found on both the tops and soles of the feet. On the tops of the feet they are located between the diaphragm and waist lines. The reflex points covering those parts of the lymphatic system (see p.95) that are found in the upper half of the body (that is, above the waist) are located at the base of the webs between the toes. Working reflexes across zones two and three on this part of the feet also helps treat the chest area. Additionally, the reflexes for the musculature of the ribs can be found in the area that surrounds the lung reflexes.

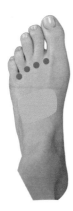
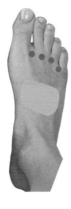

Work these reflexes in vertical strips from the webs between the toes to the base of the marked area, moving from the medial to the lateral edge of each foot. Work first on the bones of the foot, and then on the areas in between. If there are tender spots, repeat the pressures in horizontal strips, both hands working together.

Fallopian tubes, vas deferens and groin The fallopian tubes carry the ova (eggs) from the ovaries to the uterus in the female reproductive system. The vas deferens is the tube which transports the sperm from the testicle to the penis in the male reproductive system. The reflexes for these parts of the body, and for the male and female groin areas in general, are located on the tops of both feet in a band that connects both sides of the ankle bones. Reflexology treatment of these reflexes can ease tension and muscle cramps, especially during the female menstrual cycle.

To work these reflexes, support the heel with both hands and use both thumbs to apply pressure to the top of the foot, starting from the side of each ankle and working toward the middle until your thumbs meet, taking care not to pinch the skin. Repeat three times.

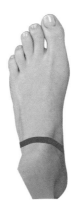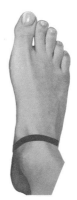

The medial (inner) side of the foot

Uterus, prostate and musculature of pelvis The reflexes for the uterus (womb) on female patients and the prostate on male patients are located on the heel in a point found at the base of the groin reflex on the medial side of the foot. For more deep-seated problems relating to the uterus and prostate, the chronic uterus and chronic prostate reflexes can be treated. These are found on the medial side of the foot, in a vertical line rising above the ankle bone. The reflex areas covering the musculature of the pelvis lie across the inner side of the heel covering quite a large area.

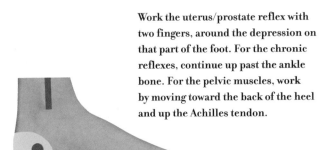

Work the uterus/prostate reflex with two fingers, around the depression on that part of the foot. For the chronic reflexes, continue up past the ankle bone. For the pelvic muscles, work by moving toward the back of the heel and up the Achilles tendon.

Spine and trachea/bronchi The various spinal reflexes, corresponding to the cervical, thoracic, lumbar, sacrum and coccyx parts of the spine, are found on the medial sides of both the feet, along the arches, in a line from the middle of the great toe to the mid-part of the heel. Applying pressure to these reflexes can help any back or leg problems. In fact, if you don't have time to give (or receive) a full reflexology treatment, spending just five minutes working on the spine area is a great first-aid treatment for someone who is feeling a little unwell. The reflexes for the trachea (windpipe) and the bronchi (the main airways into the lungs) are found on the inner side of the great toe, just below the base of the nail.

Work the spine reflexes by applying pressure with the thumb along the whole of the arch of the foot. Travel from heel to toe and continue along to the trachea/bronchi reflex, before changing direction. You can also work any of the individual areas in short vertical strips. Repeat several times.

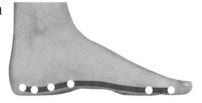

The lateral (outer) side of the foot

Shoulder and axillary areas A key reflex point for the complex part of the body that is the shoulder is found between the shoulder line and the diaphragm line (see p.25) on the lateral side and soles of both feet. See also the reflex map of the tops of the feet (p.123) for the reflex area covering the shoulder muscle, which lies at the base of the third, fourth and fifth toes. The reflexes for the axillary (armpit) area of the body continue from the shoulder reflex, round and under the foot, on the bottom of the fourth and fifth toes and down to the diaphragm line.

Work along the lateral side of the foot from the fifth toe to the diaphragm line. Repeat several times. Next, work in diagonal strips on the area from the third, fourth and fifth toes to the diaphragm line, on the tops and soles of the feet.

Chronic sciatic, ovaries and testes, musculature of buttocks The reflex for the ovaries in female patients and the testes in male patients is located at the base of the groin reflex on the lateral side of both feet. It is surrounded by the reflex area for the musculature of the buttocks, which covers quite a large area. The chronic sciatic reflex is found on the lateral side of the foot in a vertical line rising above the outer edge of the ankle bone. In addition, if you continue working toward the back of the heel and up the Achilles tendon at the back of the ankle you will find the reflexes that cover the general musculature of the spinal area.

The ovaries/testes reflex and buttocks reflex area are worked in exactly the same way as the uterus/prostate and pelvic, but on the lateral aspect of the heel. Continue up to work the chronic sciatic reflex, above the ankle bone, up and down in a vertical line.

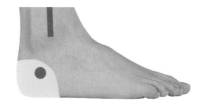

Hips, knees and elbows There is one reflex area on the lateral aspect of the left foot to cover the knee and elbow on the left-hand side of the body, and another reflex area in the same place on the right foot to cover the knee and the elbow on the right-hand side of the body. They are located on the lateral side of each foot, on the waist line (see p.25) and around the "notch" that you can feel in the middle of the lateral edge of the foot. The reflex area for another of the body's complicated joints, the hip, is found in a crescent-shaped area underneath the outer ankle bone on each foot.

For the knee and elbow reflex, work in vertical lines over the bony area in the middle of the lateral edge with two fingers or your thumb. Work upward to treat the elbow, and downward to treat the knee. To treat the hip reflex, slightly elevate the foot and work back and forth along the area several times.

Completing the session

When you have finished treating the different reflexes of the feet, end the session by performing a couple of relaxation techniques. Apply firm, unmoving pressure to the solar plexus points (see p.51), while the patient inhales and exhales slowly and deeply. Try also the "spinal twist" technique: place both hands on the medial edge of the spinal reflex, with your thumbs on the sole of the foot and your fingers lying across the top. Hold the hand nearest to the ankle stationary, and move the hand nearest to the toes back and forth two or three times.

Once you have finished the reflexology part of the session, apply foot lotion and massage the feet – a highly relaxing and enjoyable part of the treatment. Use your knuckles on the heel area, and your fist on the sole of the foot, sweeping down from the toes to the heel area. Continue right up to the knee.

Congratulations! Whether you have been treating yourself or another person, you will have just completed a holistic treatment of great benefit to the physical and emotional health and well-being of the recipient.

BASIC FOOT CARE

Taking care of the feet is vitally important, but often it is something overlooked by many people. The feet suffer so much wear and tear just as a result of everyday living. However, by following some basic foot-care tips and performing some simple foot exercises, you can maintain good foot health and make a positive impact on your health and well-being generally.

Give yourself a weekly pedicure at home to help minor foot ailments and provide your feet with a well-deserved treat. Soak your feet in warm water for about ten minutes. Dry them thoroughly, especially between the toes, and then apply a good moisturiser that penetrates quickly. This will soften any calloused areas and help remove dead cells, revealing smoother skin. It will also help to treat dry, cracked or itchy skin between the toes. If this persists, however, seek medical advice as it could indicate a fungal infection. Trim toenails straight across to minimize the risk of any ingrowing, which can be extremely painful in the affected area and can also cause headaches. Finally, make sure you wear shoes that have a generous toe box and do not squeeze your feet.

The following easy foot exercises keep the feet supple and energize the body by boosting the circulation. They also have the added advantage of gently stimulating certain reflex areas which, in turn, have a beneficial effect on the corresponding body parts.

- Wriggle your toes and splay them out – this helps loosen them and also helps remedy neck and head problems.
- Rotate each foot both ways, making a large circle with the great toe, pointing it first to the floor then to the ceiling – this helps the hip and spine area.
- Pick up a pen off the floor with your toes – this also helps your neck.
- For tired or aching legs, place a rolled-up towel under one foot and, holding both ends, pull it up toward while trying to straighten the leg – this also aids the back.
- Place any round object, such as a golf or tennis ball, under your foot and roll from toe to heel and back again – this also helps to stimulate all the internal reflexes.

Heaven is under our feet
as well as over our heads.

HENRY DAVID THOREAU

(1817–62)

The light of the sun and the moon
illuminates the whole world,
both him who does well and him who does ill,
both him who stands high and him who stands low.

THE BUDDHA

(c.563–c.483BCE)

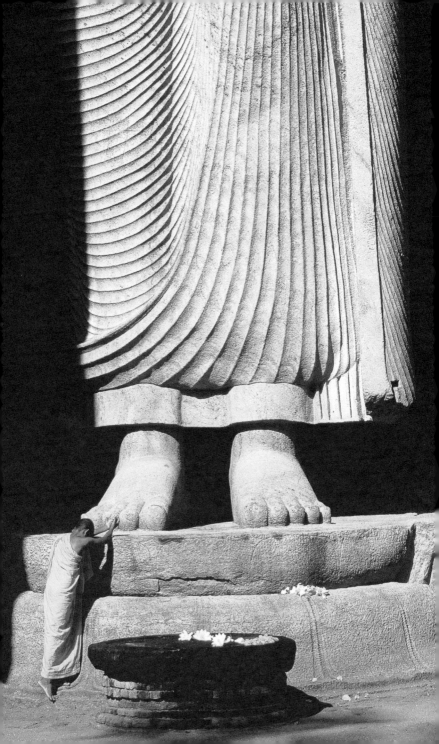

hand reflexology

Like the feet, the hands are structurally intricate but they also have amazing dexterity. They contain literally thousands of nerve endings, hence the great sensitivity of the fingertips. Our minds and hands work in close unison at all times. When we are cold we rub our hands automatically – this warms and stimulates the circulation, helping to maintain our health.

Reflexology applied to the hands is a milder, gentler alternative to treating the feet as the reflex points are not quite as powerful and treatment doesn't stimulate the release of as many toxins around the body as foot reflexology. As such, it is particularly suitable for vulnerable groups such as the very young, the elderly or the terminally ill. It remains, however, highly effective in rebalancing body systems, easing tension and boosting general health and well-being. Hand reflexology is easy to do, on yourself as well as on others, and is well worth incorporating into your daily routine. Reflex points on the hands can be worked frequently without any undue side effects.

In this chapter we present a basic reflexology session for the hands. We discuss various interpreting and holding techniques, and show you how to warm and relax the hands before starting treatment. This is followed by a step-by-step hand reflexology session that will treat the whole body.

INTERPRETING THE HAND

Like the feet, the hands are windows through which the health of the whole body can be seen. Before giving a hand-reflexology treatment, take time to look carefully at your patient's hands so that you can identify any potential problem areas on which to focus during the session. Take account, too, of the person's demeanour when they arrive (see pp.44–5), and tailor your work according to your complete analysis.

A person's nails will tell you the most about their health. For example, research has shown that many glandular problems and endocrine disorders result in malfunction of the nail growth. Examine the nails with the following criteria in mind:

• Nails should be pink and healthy, and, when pressed, their colour should return quickly. Pale nails indicate a systemic disorder, such as of the circulatory system.
• White marks or flecks on the nails often indicate some trauma or illness. It takes about six months for a nail to

grow from its base to its tip. Observing the position of the mark or fleck will give a good indication of when the problem took place.

- If the patient suffers from an iron deficiency the nails will often be concave, or spoon-shaped.
- Ridged lines on the nails (called Beaus Lines) often indicate some kind of respiratory disorder.
- Nails that take on an exaggerated curvature (called Hippocratic nails) may also signal a respiratory disorder or a thyroid imbalance.

Also check for any of the following signs:

- Blue areas on the hands or nails. This may indicate poor circulation and, if they appear on the padded area of the thumb joint, could signal a stomach problem.
- Yellow areas on the hands or nails. These are owing to high levels of toxins in the body and are often evident in smokers or those who consume alcohol to excess.
- Fingers that lean rather than being straight. These can indicate a problem in the corresponding zonal area of the neck.

HOLDING THE HAND

You can use several supporting and holding techniques during a session of hand reflexology. However, no set rules apply – one hand works while the other supports, using the technique that you and your patient find most comfortable and that gives you the best access to the reflexes you wish to work during the session.

1   Perhaps the most common hold is "shaking hands" which can be used to work easily on most areas of the hand.

2   When working on your patient's palm, let their hand rest gently on your upturned palm. Interlock your thumb with theirs to hold the hand in position.

3   When working on the top of the hand, hold your patient's fingers in a slightly bent position, to give a flat working surface with no creases.

4   When working on the sides of the hands or the fingers, hold the hand in a vertical position, encircling most of it with your supporting hand.

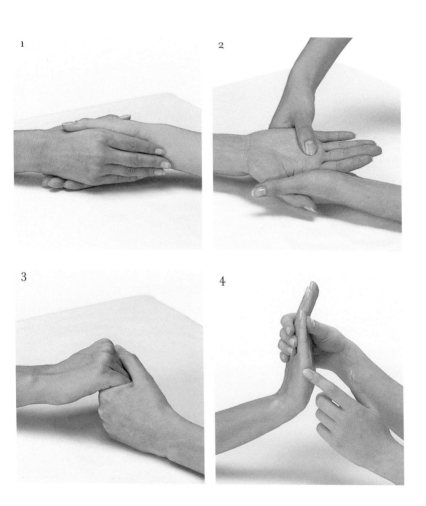

A BASIC SESSION FOR THE HANDS

This section presents a basic reflexology session for the hands. We begin with some warming and relaxing techniques before practising the step-by-step treatment.

Warming and relaxing techniques

These techniques can be repeated at intervals during the session, changing hands as required.

1 **Stroking** Supporting the hand, palm up, with your left hand, push down into the palm with your fingers, then draw them along the palm to the finger tips.

2 **Flexing** Interlock fingers with your patient, right hand to right hand, with your left hand supporting their arm. Flex the hand back and forth, and rotate the wrist.

3 **Side-to-side relaxation** Interlock your thumbs with the thumb and little finger of your patient's hand, with their palm facing you. Move your hands backward and forward.

4 **Hand moulding** Interlock your right thumb with your patient's right thumb, palm to palm, in upright position. Mould and roll the hand between both of your palms.

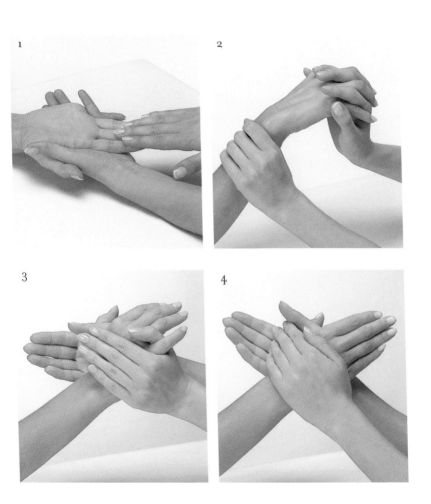

Working on the hands

Work on the right hand first, and then the left. See also the maps on pages 120–21 to locate the reflex points.

1   Support the hand, palm upward, with both of your hands. Using deep pressure with both thumbs, make small circular movements over the whole surface. This improves circulation and oxygenates the cells.

2   Using your right hand support the patient's right hand, palm upward. Work from the little finger, pulling the

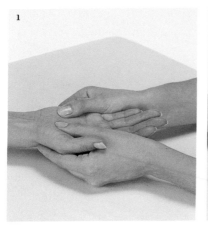
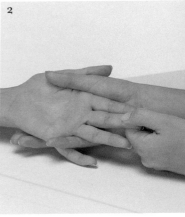

whole length of each finger and the thumb. Rotate each finger in both directions. This stimulates the brain and neck areas and helps work the eye, ear and sinus reflexes.

3 Continue to work all of these reflexes by using your thumb and index finger to apply alternating pressure (see p.23) over the top and palmar surfaces and both sides of each finger, going right down into webs.

4 Hold the hand in your left thumb and fingers. Support each finger in turn and use the knuckle of your index finger to work on the tips to boost the brain reflex.

3

4

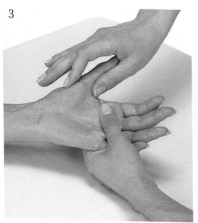
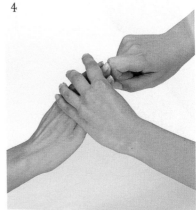

5 Return to a "shaking hands" position (see p.78). Make a fist with your left hand and starting with the little finger grip each finger between your knuckles and pull up toward the tips. This works the neck and shoulder reflexes.

6 Using both your thumbs work on either side of your patient's fingers. In particular rotate on the eye reflex (second finger, between the first joint and the tip), and the ear reflex (third finger, between the first joint and the tip).

7 Support the patient's right hand with your left, palms up, and work the lung area on the pads beneath the fingers.

5

6

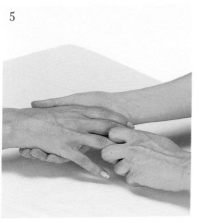
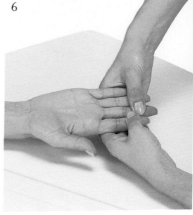

Work back and forth across the area, changing support as needed. This aids the circulation and promotes relaxation.

8 Support the patient's palm from underneath with all your fingers. Stretch their palm as much as possible, and press and knead it with your thumbs. This covers the reflexes to the digestive and intestinal tracts, and the urinary system. Increase pressure gently on sore spots. Stimulation will make the palm quite red as cellular activity increases. Continue around the base of the palm and the outside edge of the thumb for lumbar areas.

7

8

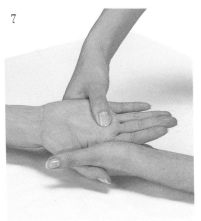
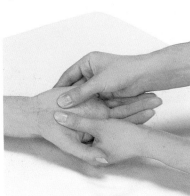

9   Ask your patient to turn their hand over and make a loose fist. Support underneath with your fingers, and work your thumbs over the top of the hand to stimulate reflexes to the lungs and abdominal organs.

10   In the same position use alternating pressure on the metacarpal bones (found between the wrist and the fingers) and between them, on the top of the hand. Also work between the webs for the lymphatics, shoulder and arm areas, and to relax the the tendons of the hand. Repeat all moves on the left hand.

9
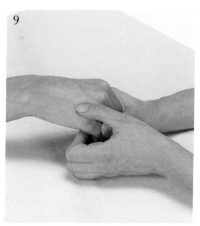

10
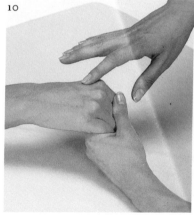

Completing the session

Finish the treatment by applying some good-quality hand cream and massaging the hands all over. Work with your thumbs over the patient's hands and up the wrists and forearms, sweeping and pressing in circular movements. Work up the bones of each forearm (the radius and ulna) to stimulate the localized nerve endings and increase the circulation of the blood, then work up the middle of each forearm. Interlock your hand with your patient's hand (see p.81, step 2) and shake gently two or three times.

It is not until someone has had a reflexology treatment and massage on the hands that they realise just what a relaxing experience it can be. Applying pressure to the hand reflexes really can benefit the whole body: the corresponding organs and systems are stimulated to work optimally, circulation is improved and muscles relax, easing tension and inducing a state of great calm.

Also, hand reflexology is so easy to perform on yourself that I thoroughly recommend a daily treatment to improve your general health and well-being, not least by relieving everyday stress and tension.

To what shall
I liken the world?
Moonlight, reflected
In dew-drops.
Shaken from a crane's bill.

DOGEN

(1200–1253)

Every dew-drop and rain-drop had
a whole heaven within it.

HENRY WADSWORTH LONGFELLOW

(1807–1882)

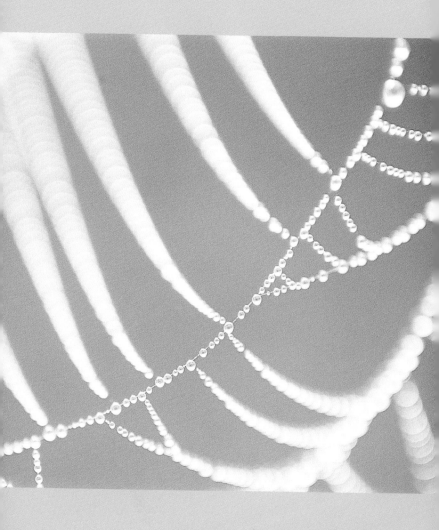

the next level

Reflexology is a powerful tool in the promotion and maintainance of the good health that many of us take for granted. However, it is when used as a treatment to help specific ailments and disorders that it often achieves the most remarkable results.

When you have completed a basic reflexology session on the feet or hands, whether your own or somebody else's, you may want to take the treatment to another level. In this chapter we show you how you can tailor reflexology to the specific needs of any individual. Whether they need some additional treatment to support a particular body system, such as the respiratory or cardiovascular system, or help to alleviate the symptoms of a common ailment, or require special care because they are very young, elderly or chronically ill, we discuss how best to approach this, and give information on which reflexes to treat and some of the benefits you can expect.

We are all aware of the fundamentals of keeping healthy, such as good diet, sufficient exercise and restful sleep. Adding reflexology to this mix, and making it a regular part of life, enhances a healthy lifestyle, encouraging the body's innate healing abilities and promoting the optimum function of all its parts. It is a therapy suited to all age groups that can be adapted to accomodate any special health needs.

TREATMENT FOR THE BODY SYSTEMS

The body's organs are grouped into "body systems", treatment of which can alleviate symptoms of illness and help to improve a range of ailments associated with that specific system. Once you have completed a basic foot- or hand-reflexology session, you may wish to revisit reflexes relating to a certain body system, either to help a patient's pre-existing condition, or to work on a congested reflex or sore spot that you have identified during the general treatment. See the reflex maps on pages 120–24 at the back of this book to locate the suggested reflexes (for both the feet and the hands) you will need to work for each body system.

Skin, hair and nails

Together, the skin, hair and nails form the integumentary system, which acts as our bodies' first line of defence against any other organism that may harm or infect us. It is also involved in the regulation of the body's temperature. Treatment of this system helps to balance any over-secretion of the hormones and sebaceous glands in acne sufferers, and calms the production of histamine and serotonin, which are released when the skin suffers any inflammation or allergic response. By paying particular attention to the reflexes that correspond to the parts of this body system, the common ailments of acne, eczema and skin allergies can be improved. To help this body system, work on the thyroid, brain and pituitary reflexes.

The respiratory system

This body system comprises all the organs involved in the breathing process, from the nose, sinuses and throat, down the windpipe to the lungs, diaphragm and intercostal muscles. Reflexology treatment clears congestion by reducing the production of excessive amounts of mucus. It also calms inflammation and aids breathing. Working on the reflexes associated with this system may help improve ailments such as asthma, bronchitis, coughs and colds, sore throats, emphysema, hay fever, sinusitis and heavy snoring. To help this body system, work on the brain, lung and intestine reflexes.

The digestive system

The mouth, oesophagus, stomach, intestines and rectum are the main organs of this system, supplemented by the liver, gall bladder and pancreas, which perform many enzyme functions involved in the digestive process. Reflexology treatment will encourage the production of digestive juices, and stimulate the absorption of nutrients. Deep relaxation during treatment also aids the whole course of digestion in general. Working the reflexes associated with this system may help alleviate acid indigestion, irritable bowel syndrome and constipation. Work on the brain, liver and pancreas reflexes.

The cardiovascular system

This system comprises the heart and its valves, the blood and blood vessels. It pumps the blood around the body, oxygenating all our tissues. A basic reflexology session will improve the circulation by stimulating the nerves, thus improving the transport of vital nutrients and hormones around the body. In addition, working the reflexes specifically associated with this system can help combat the effects of arteriosclerosis and its associated problems. More serious heart conditions should be treated only if the patient is stable, and with the agreement of their doctor. The best reflexes to work this body system more deeply are the brain, heart and adrenal reflexes.

The lymphatic system

Comprising the spleen, thymus, tonsils, adenoids, lymph nodes, vessels and ducts, this body system is another circulatory system around which the clear liquid lymph transports antibodies, cleanses cells and removes bacteria. Reflexology treatment can boost the production of lymphocytes (key cells in the body's immune response) and clear congestion or obstruction in the lymphatic vessels. Working the associated reflexes can help the body fight conditions such as anaemia, oedema and lymphoma. It will also stimulate the thymus – a vital part of the immune response system, especially important in babies and young children. To help the lymphatic system, work on the reflexes for the spleen, thymus and lymphatics.

The urinary system

The kidneys, ureters, bladder and urethra make up this body system which cleanses the blood and removes waste products via urine. Reflexology treatment can improve bladder function and the filtering action of the kidneys. This will help to stabilize blood pressure or fluid retention and balance acid and alkaline levels. It can also help improve related problems such as cystitis, urethritis, incontinence and renal colic. To help the urinary system, work on the bladder reflex first, followed by the reflexes for the ureters, kidneys and adrenal glands.

The reproductive system

In men this system comprises the testes, prostate, vas deferens and penis, and, in women, the mammary glands, ovaries, ova, uterus, fallopian tubes and vagina. Together these organs are responsible for every aspect of human reproduction. Reflexology treatment helps reduce any inflammation in the reproductive tracts, stimulating and balancing hormonal activity. For women, reflexology may relieve cramping during menstruation.

Reflexology can help with menstrual, menopausal and pelvic inflammatory problems, post natal depression, mastitis, endometriosis, prostate disorders and impotence. It can be of great benefit during pregnancy and labour but, in these cases, should be applied only by a qualified practitioner. To help this body system, work on the reflexes for the pituitary, brain, ovaries and testes.

The endocrine system

This is a system of glands that secretes the hormones responsible for most of our bodily functions directly into the bloodstream. It comprises the pituitary, hypothalamus, pineal, thyroid, thymus and adrenal glands. Treatment balances and regulates the complex actions of the hormones so that they function optimally. It also boosts the immune system in the very young, reduces inflammation and influences carbohydrate metabolism. To help this body system, work on the pituitary, thyroid and hypothalamus reflexes. Associated ailments that can be helped by reflexology include menstrual disorders, thyroid imbalance and Addison's and Cushing's diseases.

The nervous system

This body system, comprising the brain, spinal cord, and nerves, detects and interprets changes taking place in the body, and reacts by bringing about the necessary bodily action. It works with the endocrine system assisting in the regulation of many body processes. Treatment acts as general first aid to the nervous system which interplays with all of the senses (sight, hearing, smell, taste and touch), through its myriad connections to all parts and functions of the body. Work on the brain, spine and endocrinal reflexes to help the nervous system. Ailments that may benefit from this include neuralgia, sciatica, Parkinson's disease and multiple sclerosis.

The musculature

This system comprises all of the voluntary and involuntary muscles of the body. Muscle tissue consists of bundles of specialized cells that can contract, convert energy from chemical reactions into mechanical energy, and contribute to the internal heat of the body, the movement of the skeleton and posture. Treatment of the musculature reflexes can help relieve muscle spasm or cramp and reduce inflammation. It encourages relaxation of all the muscles, ligaments and tendons, easing strains and sprains. Common associated ailments that reflexology may help include muscular rheumatism, fibrositis and muscle injury. Work on the brain, spine and endocrinal reflexes to help this system.

The skeleton

All of the body's bones, bone marrow, joints, cartilage and ligaments make up the skeleton, a mobile framework which supports and protects the organs. Bones are also active, living structures involved in the production of blood cells and the storage of essential minerals. Reflexology treatment is aimed at aiding any degenerative change in the skeleton, especially arthritic disorders where it can reduce pain, inflammation and excess heat in joints. Related ailments that reflexology may help include inflammation of any joint, gout, back pain or a prolapsed disk, and spinal problems in general. Work on the spinal and adrenal reflexes to help the skeleton.

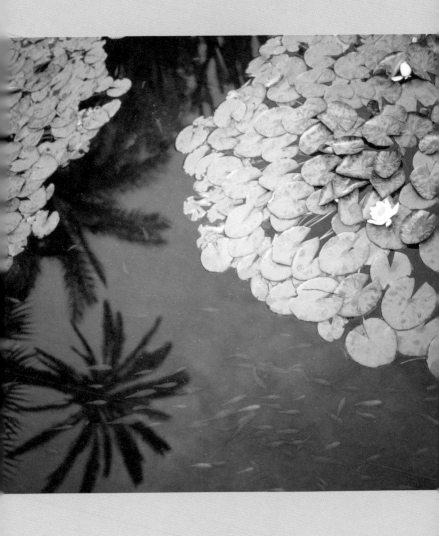

Water which is too pure has no fish.

THE TS'AI KEN T'AN

(MING DYNASTY: 1368– 1644)

Wisdom is like a clear, cool pool –
it can be entered from any side.

NAGARJUNA

(*c.*150– 250CE)

ADDRESSING COMMON AILMENTS

As discussed in previous chapters, reflexology works by rebalancing the organs and systems of the body, and stimulating them to work to optimum effect. As such, it does not actually treat a specific disorder or ailment, but facilitates the conditions in which the body can best heal itself. However, complementing a general reflexology treatment with additional work on particular areas will often produce a marked improvement in the symptoms of many common illnesses. Indeed, countless inspiring case histories testify to the disappearance of symptoms, especially pain, after a course of reflexology treatment.

The following conditions have been chosen because they represent the most common complaints appearing in my case load over many years. In each example, the condition is summarized and advice given on how best to treat it using reflexology, often with an image showing how to work a suitable reflex on either the foot or hand. As with other suggested treatments in this book, refer to the charts on pages 120–24 for precise reflex locations.

Repetitive strain injury

A very common ailment afflicting many people in the modern developed world, repetitive strain injury (RSI), in its simplest terms, is the overuse of a particular part of the body, caused by doing something too many times, often incorrectly. It is imperative to address the root cause of the problem, be it playing a particular sport, such as tennis or golf; knitting; gardening; or simply poor behavioural habits such as watching television with the neck slightly turned or sitting badly at a desk. Any of these activities can overstretch a muscle or ligament, or inflame a bony prominence, which in turn can lead to injury or damage and a great deal of pain.

To treat RSI with reflexology, begin with a full basic session and then work on the reflex that is associated with the problem area, for example the elbow or neck. If the patient's hands are badly affected, work the cross reflexes (see p.22), in this case on the feet. Also pay particular attention to the adrenal gland reflex, which is a powerful aid to any inflammatory problem, whether tendon- or muscle-related.

Skin problems

Reflexology can be highly effective in the treatment of skin complaints and is particularly helpful for the skin problems suffered by many teenagers during puberty. The relaxed state induced by a general treatment session helps equip the body to fight even the most chronic skin disorder and, coupled with a sensible diet and exercise regime, additional work on certain reflexes will significantly improve the condition in a short space of time.

The main reflexes to work are the pituitary and thyroid (shown on the foot, opposite), which helps the skin, hair and nails. Treat the liver reflex gently – it may be tender if there are any excess toxins in the body. Stimulate the adrenal gland reflex to reduce inflammation. Reflexology will improve the circulation generally so that all of the skin cells get a fresh supply of oxygen and nutrients.

Lumbago (backache)

Lower back pain combined with difficulty moving are classic symptoms of lumbago. Restriction often comes on quite suddenly, usually caused by twisting, bending or over-stretching. Reflexology, combined with careful attention to posture, can greatly improve symptoms and act as a powerful pain-reliever.

Work from the tip of the little finger down to the heel of the hand (shown on the hand, below), round to the base of the thumb and up to the tip. This covers the spinal reflex and many reflexes of associated areas, such as the neck, shoulders and hips. Also work the powerful spinal reflexes on the feet if possible. Treat the brain reflexes to stimulate production of endorphins (pain-relievers).

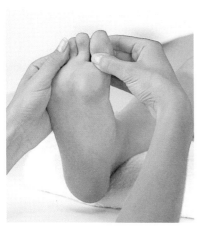
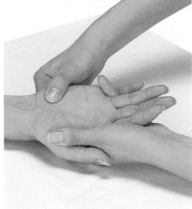

Headaches

Headaches are often caused by emotional stress or extreme fatigue, and sometimes certain foods can act as triggers. The pain we experience usually comes from the connective tissues, blood vessels and muscles of the scalp, which surround the brain.

Work the liver reflex across the middle of the foot (see foot, opposite) to help eliminate toxins from the body. Reflexology on the fingers relaxes and acts as a sedative – it also has an antispasmodic action on the muscles of the neck and scalp, stimulates the cerebral circulation and tones up the central nervous system. Also work the trigeminal nerve reflex (on the inner side of the thumb nail or the top of the great toe), which serves the whole head area. However, always have persistent headaches checked, in case of any abnormalities.

Sinusitis

Sinuses are the narrow, hollow cavities within the bones of the face and skull. They lighten the weight of the head and lend resonance to the voice. Sinusitis occurs when the mucous membrane and tiny blood vessels become infected and inflamed, making the head feel heavy with pain in the facial area.

Treat sinusitis by working all the fingers thoroughly (see below, right). This helps to rebalance the nervous system, stimulating it to act as a decongestant to relieve nasal secretions and reduce swelling. Work the liver area to combat any excess toxins in the system. Also apply extra pressure on the adrenal reflexes to stimulate their anti-inflammatory properties.

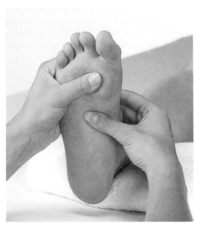
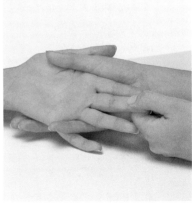

Stiff neck

A stiff neck is characterized by a severe spasm of the neck, with some restriction when moving the head. It is common for symptoms to appear on waking for no apparent reason. Possible causes might include an irritated nerve, or poor posture when sleeping, reading, watching television or holding a telephone.

To treat a stiff neck with reflexology, work the neck and cervical reflexes at the base of the thumb and first two fingers (see opposite, left). Also apply pressure to the adrenal gland reflexes to reduce inflammation, and to the brain, spinal and axillary reflexes. Work the fourth and fifth fingers from the tip to the base, then extend them gently and rotate in both directions to aid neck movement.

Digestive problems

People of all ages suffer from digestive problems from time to time in their lives. These might include constipation, indigestion, irritable bowel, diarrhoea and flatulence. Underlying causes may be anxiety or stress compounded by poor diet and lack of exercise.

After a full basic reflexology session, which will relax a tense digestive system, pay particular attention to stimulating the liver and pancreas reflexes found between the diaphragm and the waist lines on the soles and palms (see example on the palm, below right). The pancreas secretes digestive enzymes which help to break down any food eaten, and the liver processes dissolved digested products and de-toxifies the blood. Also treat the thyroid reflex, which is responsible for speeding up or slowing down the metabolic rate.

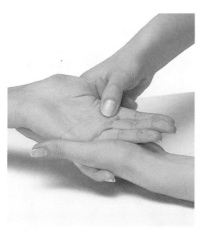
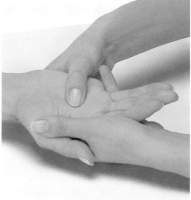

REFLEXOLOGY FOR SPECIAL CARE

The natural, holistic and non-invasive nature of reflex-ology makes it a therapy especially well-suited to certain groups, such as young children, the elderly and those suffering chronic illness. In other words, for all those who would particularly benefit from a boost to their immune systems and for whom more radical treatments may be undesirable. Reflexology can play a key role in strengthening and stimulating an immature or weak-ened immune system and, equally, can provide a strong complementary arm to support a drug-based treatment program, for example in the case of chronic illness. The treatment promotes the self-regulation of the body's internal environment, helping it to curb overactive or increase underactive bodily functions, such as enzyme secretion or hormone production.

The positive effects of reflexology for special care groups cannot be overstated. All manner of complaints that commonly affect them either because they are so young, or because age has diminished some aspects of their health or mobility, or because a chronic illness has debilitated them, leaving them physically and emotionally weak, can be treated to great effect.

This section takes a look at the three aforementioned groups in turn. It addresses some special requirements they might have and explains how reflexology can help.

Babies and young children

Gentle application of reflexology treatments on the hands and feet of infants and small children will help to strengthen their developing immune systems and provide protection against, and relief from, many of the minor but irritating problems they are prone to suffer. These might include teething, infant colic, digestive upsets and childhood fevers. However, if you think that a child is suffering from undue pain or an abnormal disturbance of any kind, the child should be referred to a medical practitioner before you try reflexology.

A peaceful and comfortable baby generally does not cry. If he (or she) does and you know he is not hungry, thirsty, too hot, too cold or in need of a nappy/diaper

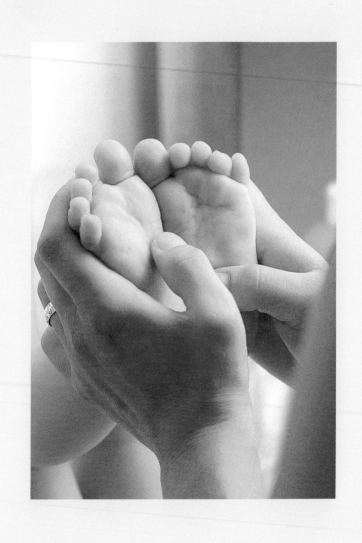

change, he may be suffering a minor complaint that can be helped with reflexology. Respond to the infant by working on some reflex points and see immediately how he will involuntarily react to your touch. As well as relieving physical symptoms that are causing distress, treating your child with reflexology creates a very strong psychological and emotional bond between the two of you.

The actions of the well-known nursery rhymes involving touch, "This little piggy went to market", and "Round and round the garden, like a teddy bear", performed on even the tiniest foot or hand, act as very gentle reflexology and can have the most profound effect of calming babies and toddlers. This is because they cover so many reflex points. This light treatment on the foot or hand will also boost a child's immune systems and work in a preventative capacity.

If your child is suffering from teething troubles, he may have red, swollen gums, disturbed sleep, no appetite and be fretful and irritable. Occasionally these symptoms are accompanied by secondary infections such as a high temperature or earache. To reduce the effects of teething problems by using reflexology, work all over the first three toes of each foot. This is where the facial reflexes are located (see pp.122–23).

For agitation and distress caused by teething or any other childhood complaint, work the area from the neck reflex down to the diaphragm line on both the hands and the feet. This area includes the thymus reflex, which is found on the inner edge of the soles of both feet, just above the diaphragm line. The thymus is a key organ in an immature immune system, responsible for stimulating the body's defences into action. Working the diaphragm reflex in this area also relaxes the breathing.

When treating babies, caress the surface of the skin only very gently. As children get older you may apply more pressure and work the area several times daily, especially when an infection is present. As well as easing distress and boosting the immune system, a gentle reflexology session will often reduce the high temperature that so commonly accompanies childhood illness.

A general treatment comprising the light stretching and rotating of all the fingers and toes will benefit children enormously as it stimulates all ten of the body zones (see p.21), boosting their health and vitality. Incorporate regular reflexology into your family's routine to help ward off illness and maintain good health.

The elderly

Aging is a natural process, which brings a decline in certain body processes, such as lung function, resistance to infection and good mobility. Blood vessels often thicken, impairing their function and restricing blood flow to vital organs around the body. Physical restrictions may also impinge on mental and emotional well-being with many people becoming much less active as they get older. Also, mental ability may decline as a result of a poor blood supply to the brain. Keeping as active as possible in later life, both physically and mentally, is key to maintaining optimum health.

As well as rebalancing and revitalizing the body's organs and systems generally, a daily basic reflexology treatment, on the hands or feet, stimulates the circulatory system, improving blood supply to the brain and boosting energy. Treatment will also help to maintain good bowel and bladder function, and reduce stiffness and joint pain caused by inflammation, thus aiding mobility. As with young children, special care should be taken when treating older patients, as their skin is thinner and less supple, and ligaments may be stiff.

Work the reflexes associated with any particular problem suffered. In addition, the adrenal gland reflex helps reduce inflammation, and the thyroid reflex benefits arthritis and the musculoskeletal system generally.

Reflexology, especially on the hands, is highly suitable for older people as it is easy to apply, totally non-invasive and offers a calming and relaxing experience, with real health benefits.

The chronically ill

Treating sufferers of chronic illness with reflexology is something that is becoming more and more widespread. Indeed, an increasing number of clinics specializing in complementary therapies such as reflexology are being set up to run in conjunction with traditional medical treatments as the developed world adopts a more holistic approach to healthcare. Such clinics treat patients suffering from a wide range of conditions including cancer, HIV/AIDS and multiple sclerosis.

While reflexology practitioners do not claim miracle cures for chronic or degenerative conditions, the clear benefits that treatment brings to the mind and body can affect sufferers only in a positive way. However, it is important always to work closely with the patient's medical team when treating chronic conditions.

A basic reflexology session, applied gently and with great sensitivity to the hands or feet, can bring benefits to someone suffering from a chronic illness that might include an improvement in general energy levels, an increase in the expulsion of toxins from the body, and a reduction in levels of pain experienced. The boost in energy levels, coupled with the deep relaxation often gained from treatment, not only helps to alleviate feelings of stress and tension but can also lead to the patient feeling able to adopt a more positive outlook on and approach to their condition.

You ask why I live
alone in the mountain forest,

and I smile and am silent
until even my soul grows quiet:

it lives in the other world,
one that no one owns.

The peach trees blossom.
The water continues to flow.

LI PO
(701–762CE)

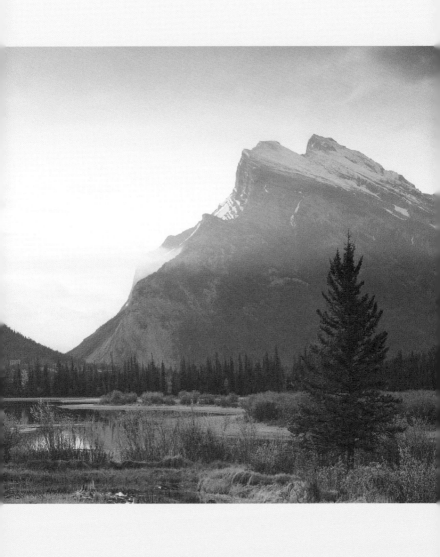

REFLEX ZONES OF THE PALMS OF THE HANDS

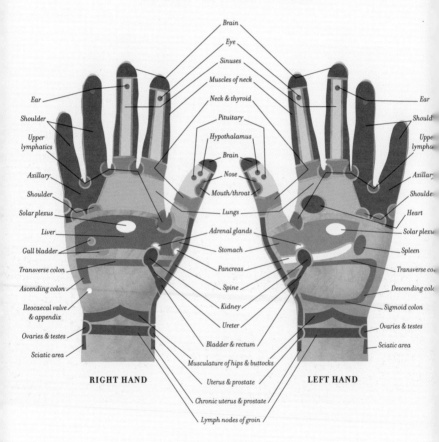

Brain
Eye
Sinuses
Muscles of neck
Neck & thyroid
Pituitary
Hypothalamus
Brain
Nose
Mouth/throat
Lungs
Adrenal glands
Stomach
Pancreas
Spine
Kidney
Ureter
Bladder & rectum
Musculature of hips & buttocks
Uterus & prostate
Chronic uterus & prostate
Lymph nodes of groin

Ear
Shoulder
Upper lymphatics
Axillary
Shoulder
Solar plexus
Liver
Gall bladder
Transverse colon
Ascending colon
Ileocaecal valve & appendix
Ovaries & testes
Sciatic area

Ear
Should
Uppe lympha
Axillar
Shoulde
Heart
Solar plexu
Spleen
Transverse co
Descending col
Sigmoid colon
Ovaries & testes
Sciatic area

RIGHT HAND

LEFT HAND

REFLEX ZONES OF THE TOPS OF THE HANDS

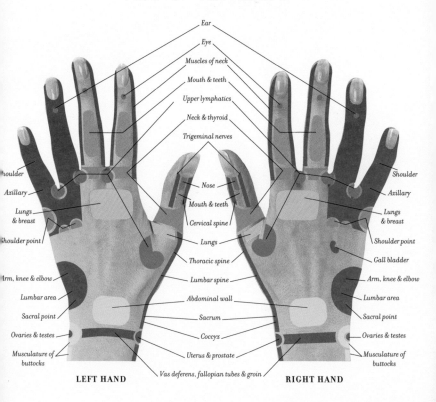

Ear
Eye
Muscles of neck
Mouth & teeth
Upper lymphatics
Neck & thyroid
Trigeminal nerves

Shoulder
Axillary
Lungs & breast
Shoulder point
Arm, knee & elbow
Lumbar area
Sacral point
Ovaries & testes
Musculature of buttocks

Shoulder
Axillary
Lungs & breast
Shoulder point
Gall bladder
Arm, knee & elbow
Lumbar area
Sacral point
Ovaries & testes
Musculature of buttocks

Nose
Mouth & teeth
Cervical spine
Lungs
Thoracic spine
Lumbar spine
Abdominal wall
Sacrum
Coccyx
Uterus & prostate
Vas deferens, fallopian tubes & groin

LEFT HAND

RIGHT HAND

REFLEX ZONES OF THE
SOLES OF THE FEET

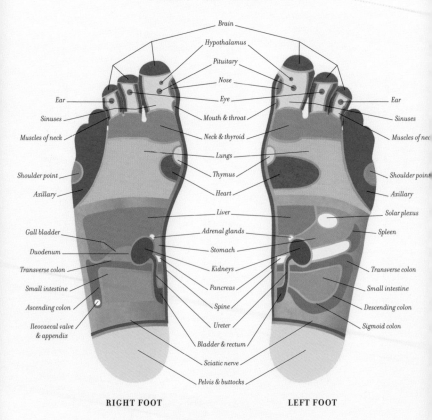

Brain
Hypothalamus
Pituitary
Nose
Ear — Eye — Ear
Sinuses — Mouth & throat — Sinuses
Muscles of neck — Neck & thyroid — Muscles of neck
Lungs
Shoulder point — Thymus — Shoulder point
Axillary — Heart — Axillary
Liver — Solar plexus
Gall bladder — Adrenal glands — Spleen
Duodenum — Stomach
Transverse colon — Kidneys — Transverse colon
Small intestine — Pancreas — Small intestine
Ascending colon — Spine — Descending colon
Ileocaecal valve — Ureter — Sigmoid colon
& appendix
Bladder & rectum
Sciatic nerve
Pelvis & buttocks

RIGHT FOOT   **LEFT FOOT**

REFLEX ZONES OF THE TOPS OF THE FEET

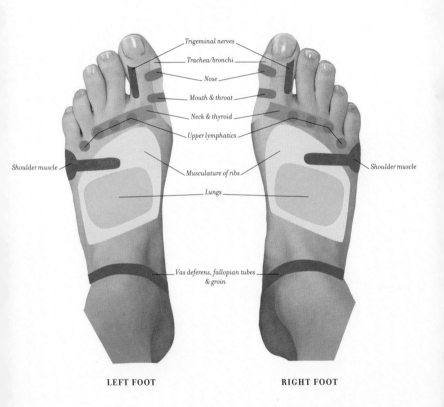

Trigeminal nerves

Trachea/bronchi

Nose

Mouth & throat

Neck & thyroid

Upper lymphatics

Shoulder muscle

Shoulder muscle

Musculature of ribs

Lungs

Vas deferens, fallopian tubes & groin

LEFT FOOT

RIGHT FOOT

REFLEX ZONES OF THE MEDIAL AND LATERAL SIDES OF THE FOOT

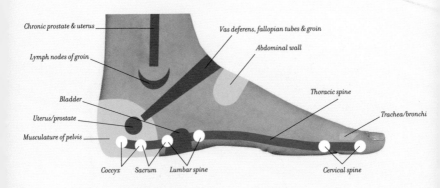

Chronic prostate & uterus

Lymph nodes of groin

Bladder

Uterus/prostate

Musculature of pelvis

Coccyx   Sacrum   Lumbar spine

Vas deferens, fallopian tubes & groin

Abdominal wall

Thoracic spine

Trachea/bronchi

Cervical spine

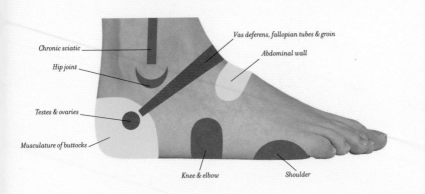

Chronic sciatic

Hip joint

Testes & ovaries

Musculature of buttocks

Knee & elbow

Shoulder

Vas deferens, fallopian tubes & groin

Abdominal wall

INDEX

Picture Credits

The publisher would like to thank the following people and photographic libraries for permission to reproduce their material. Every care has been taken to trace copyright holders. However, if we have omitted anyone we apologise and will, if informed, make corrections in any future editions.

Page 13 Werner Forman Archive; 30 Michael Holford/Victoria & Albert Museum; 41 Getty Images/Image Bank/Grant Faint; 73 Getty Images/Stone/James Strachan; 89 Digital Vision; 100 Getty Images/Stone/Victoria Pearson; 112 Photodisc; 119 Rubberball Productions

Author's Acknowledgments

Sincere thanks to everyone at DBP, especially Becky Miles, and to the models and photographic team. It was lovely working with you all and the help and guidance I received from everyone was greatly appreciated. Together we have created an inspirational and beautiful book of which we can all be proud.

Publisher's Acknowledgments

Models: Caroline Long and Suzi Langhorne
Make-up artist: Tinks Reding